SWEET DREAMS
Copyright © 2025 by DR. CHRISTOPHER J. ALLEN
Library of Congress Control Number is on file.
Hardcover ISBN: 979-8-9988989-6-9
Paperback ISBN: 979-8-9988989-5-2
eBook ISBN: 979-8-9988989-7-6
All rights reserved. No part of this publication may be reproduced, distributed, or transmitted in any form or by any means, including photocopying, recording, or other electronic or mechanical methods, without the prior written permission of the publisher or author, except in the case of brief quotations embodied in critical reviews and certain other noncommercial uses permitted by copyright law. Although every precaution has been taken to verify the accuracy of the information contained herein, the author and publisher assume no responsibility for any errors or omissions. No liability is assumed for damages that may result from the use of information contained within.

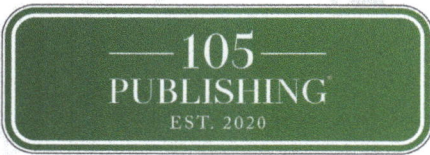

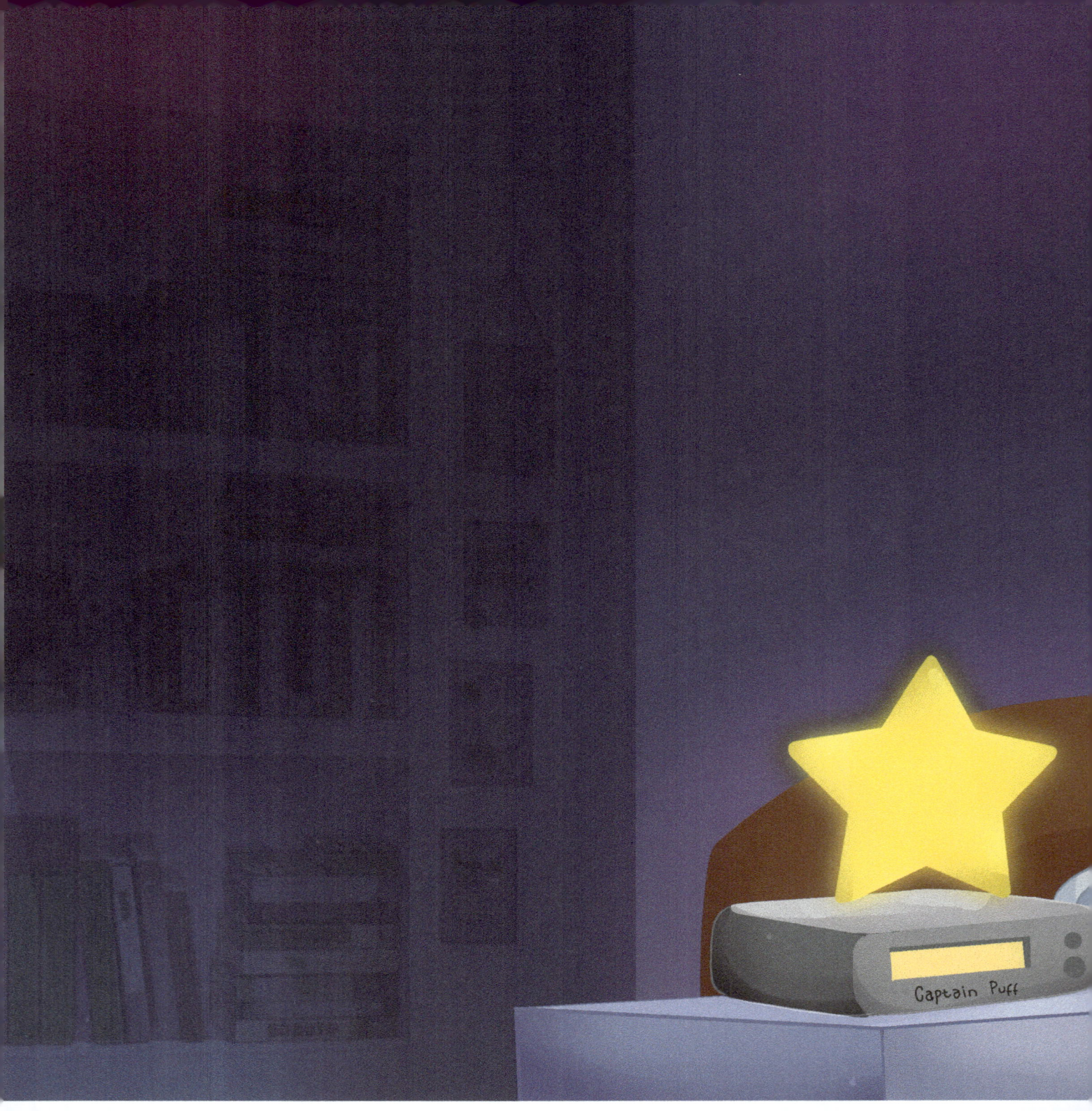

SWEET DREAMS

Written by:
Dr. Christopher J. Allen

Illustrated by:
Art Dan

*To my great-grandparents,
David and Willie Beatrice Thomas.*

Thank you for being my rock, my foundation, and my reminder that love and faith can carry generations forward.

Your quiet strength and endless encouragement shaped who I am today.

Christopher loved to help.
He helped his great-grandma read road signs on their long car rides.

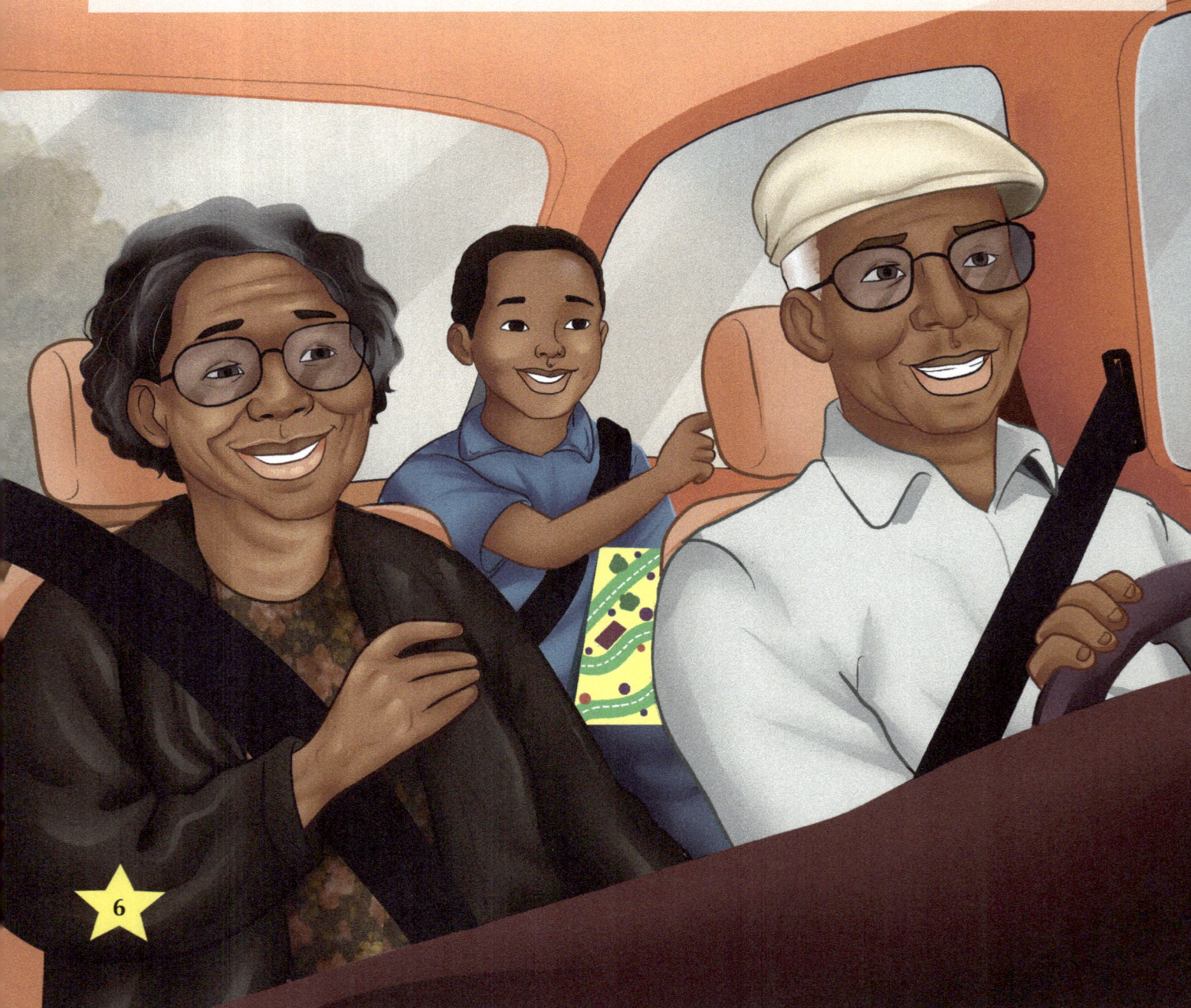

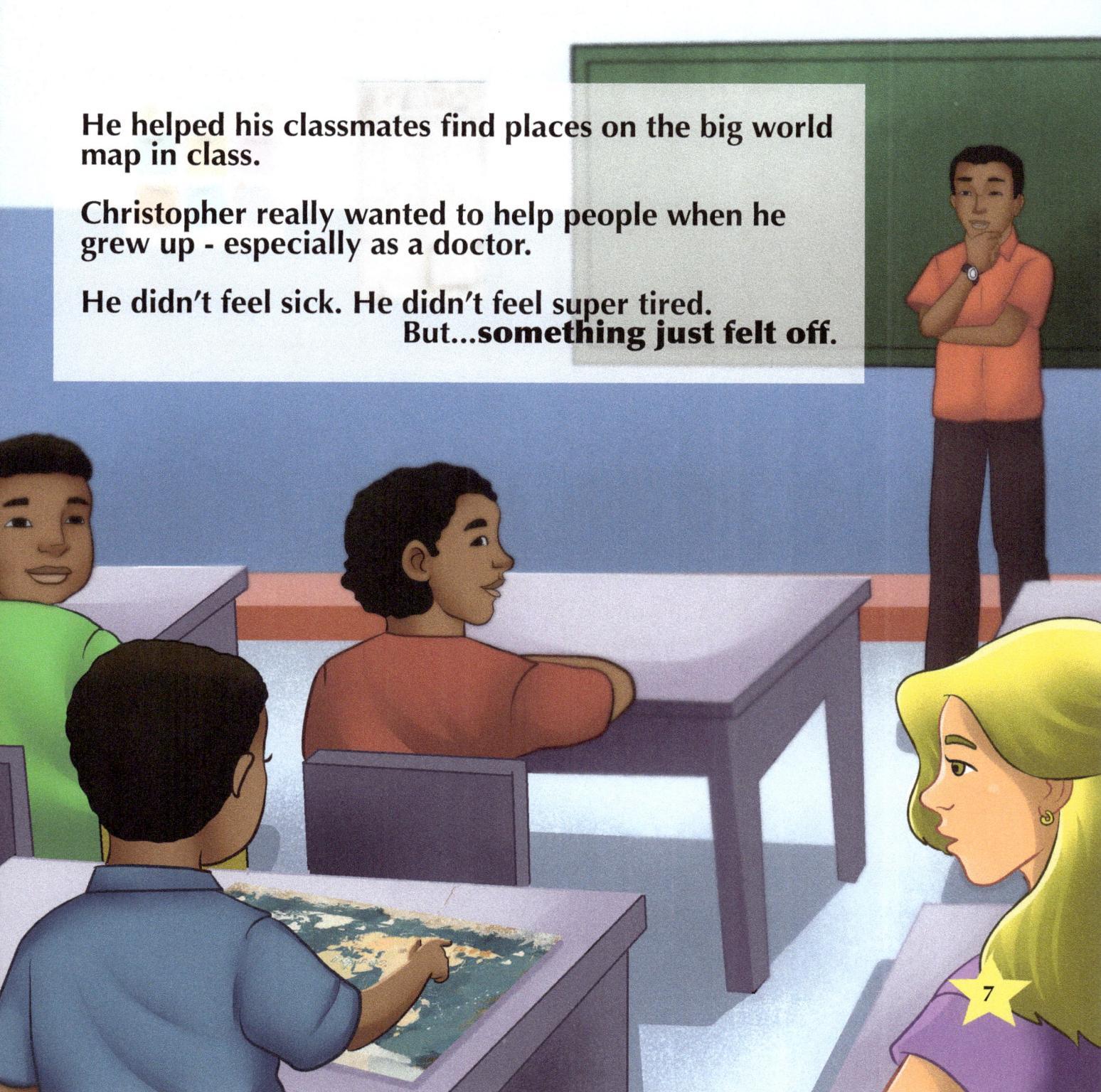

He helped his classmates find places on the big world map in class.

Christopher really wanted to help people when he grew up - especially as a doctor.

He didn't feel sick. He didn't feel super tired. But...**something just felt off**.

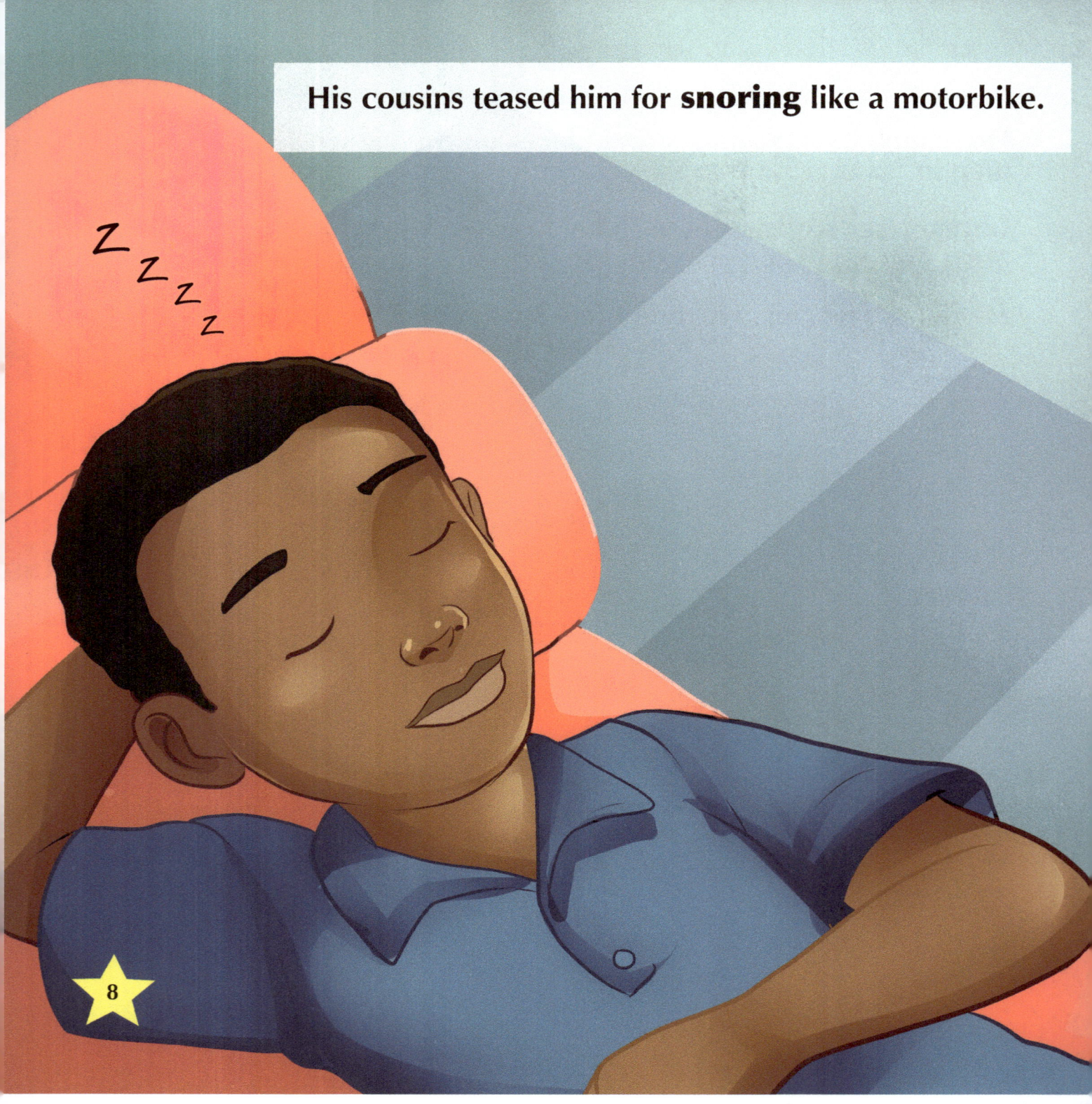

His cousins teased him for **snoring** like a motorbike.

On school trips, someone always said, "Who's making that noise?" And no matter how early he went to bed, he still yawned through math class.

Christopher wondered, "Why do I snore so loud?"

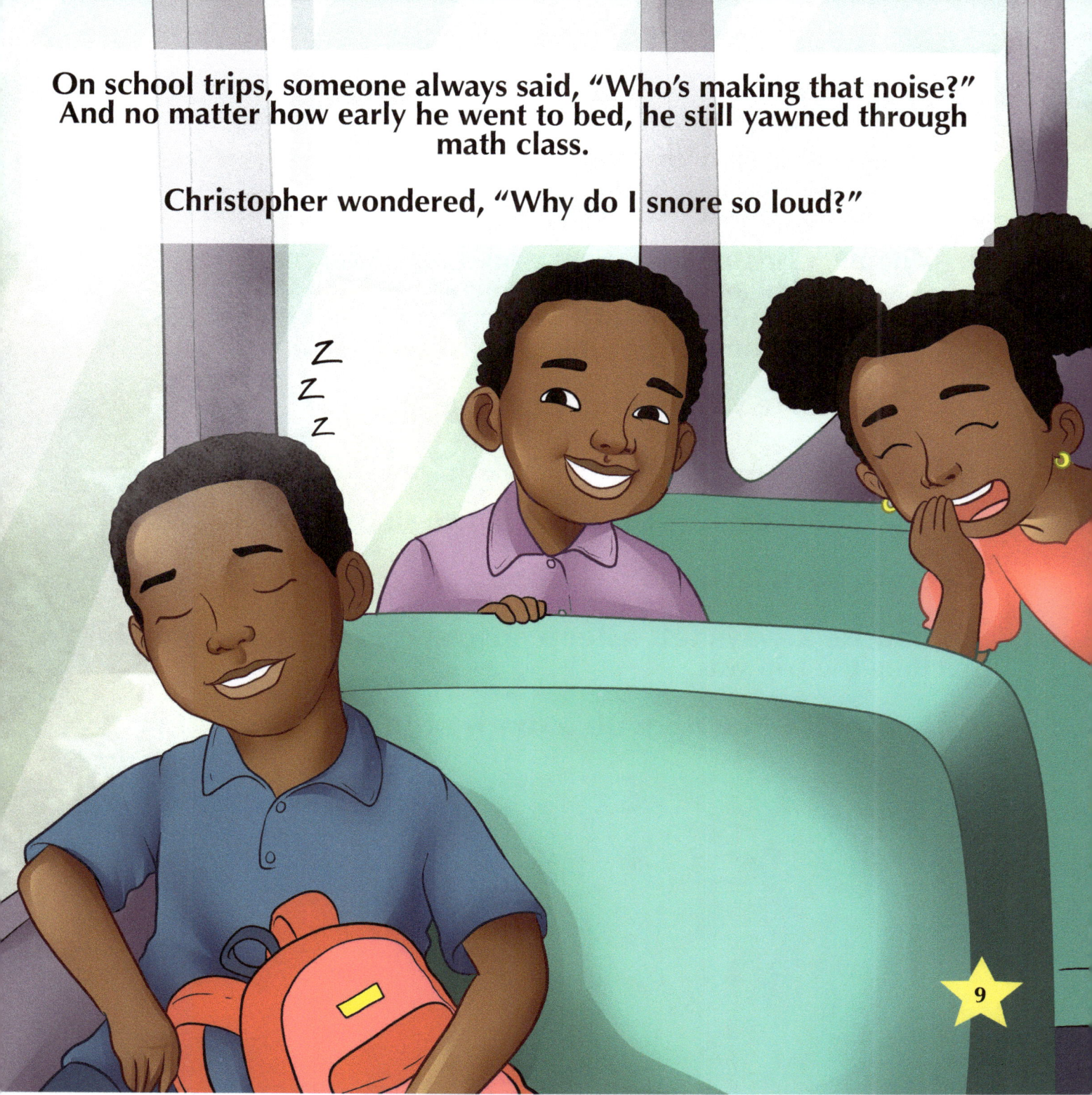

At home, Christopher's mom would peek into his room at night and hear **loud snoring** echoing down the hall.
"You sound like a little bear," she'd joke with a smile.
But sometimes, she looked more curious than amused.

"You sure you're getting good sleep, baby?" she asked.

Christopher shrugged. "I think so?"

But even he started to notice strange things...

Like how **hard** it was **to pay attention** sometimes.

Or how **he always fell asleep** on long car rides - no matter how exciting the trip was.

Or how he'd **wake up with a dry mouth and a sore throat.**

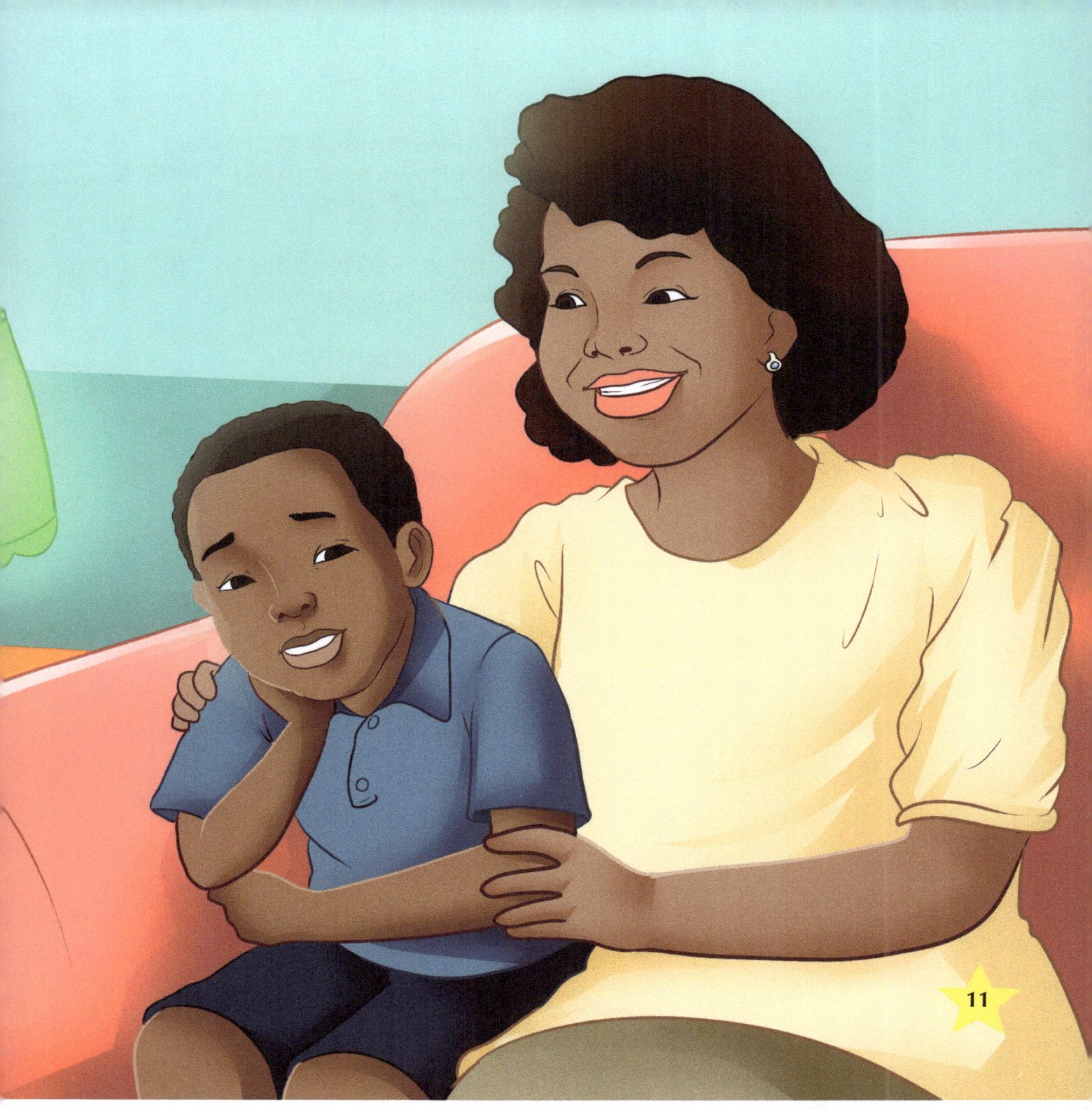

One day, something different happened at school.
A guest speaker came to the auditorium - a doctor with a stethoscope and a bright smile.

"Hi everyone! I'm Dr. Maya, and today we're going to talk about sleep." **Sleep?** Christopher's ears perked up.

The doctor pointed to a poster:
**Snoring.
Trouble paying attention.
Waking up tired.
Falling asleep in class.**

"Sometimes, these aren't just habits," she said. "They can be signs of something called **a sleep disorder**."

Christopher froze. That list? It sounded...exactly like him.

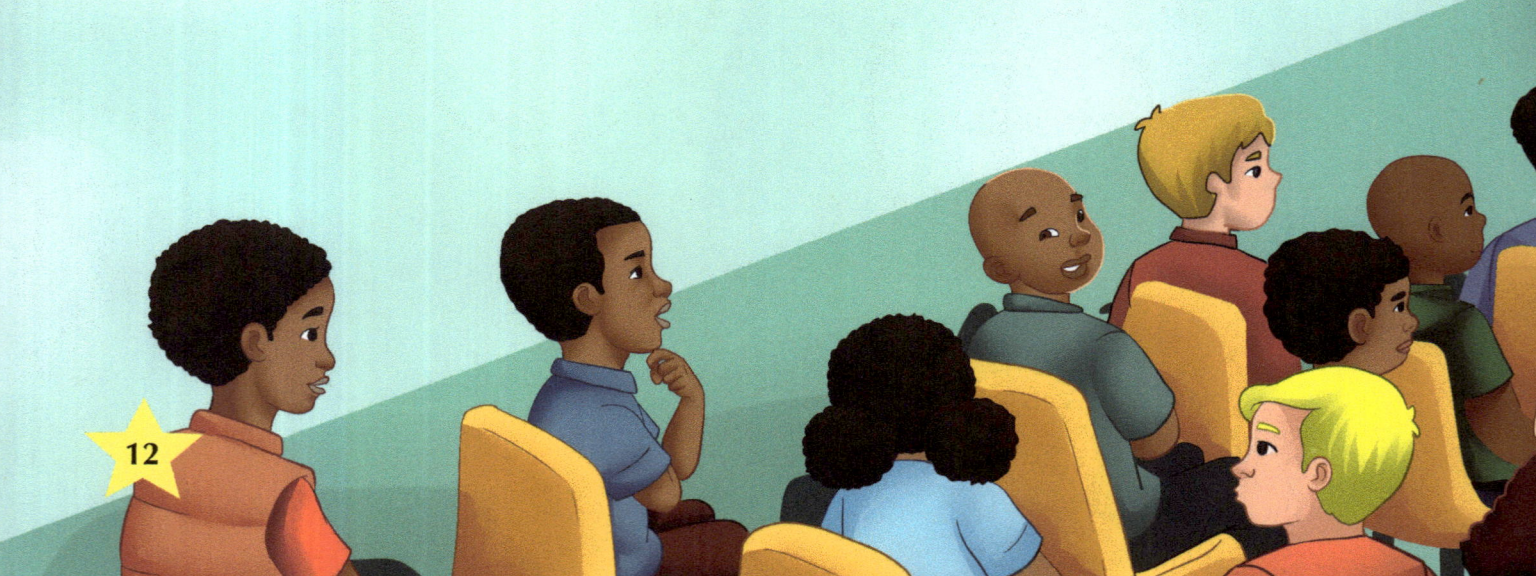

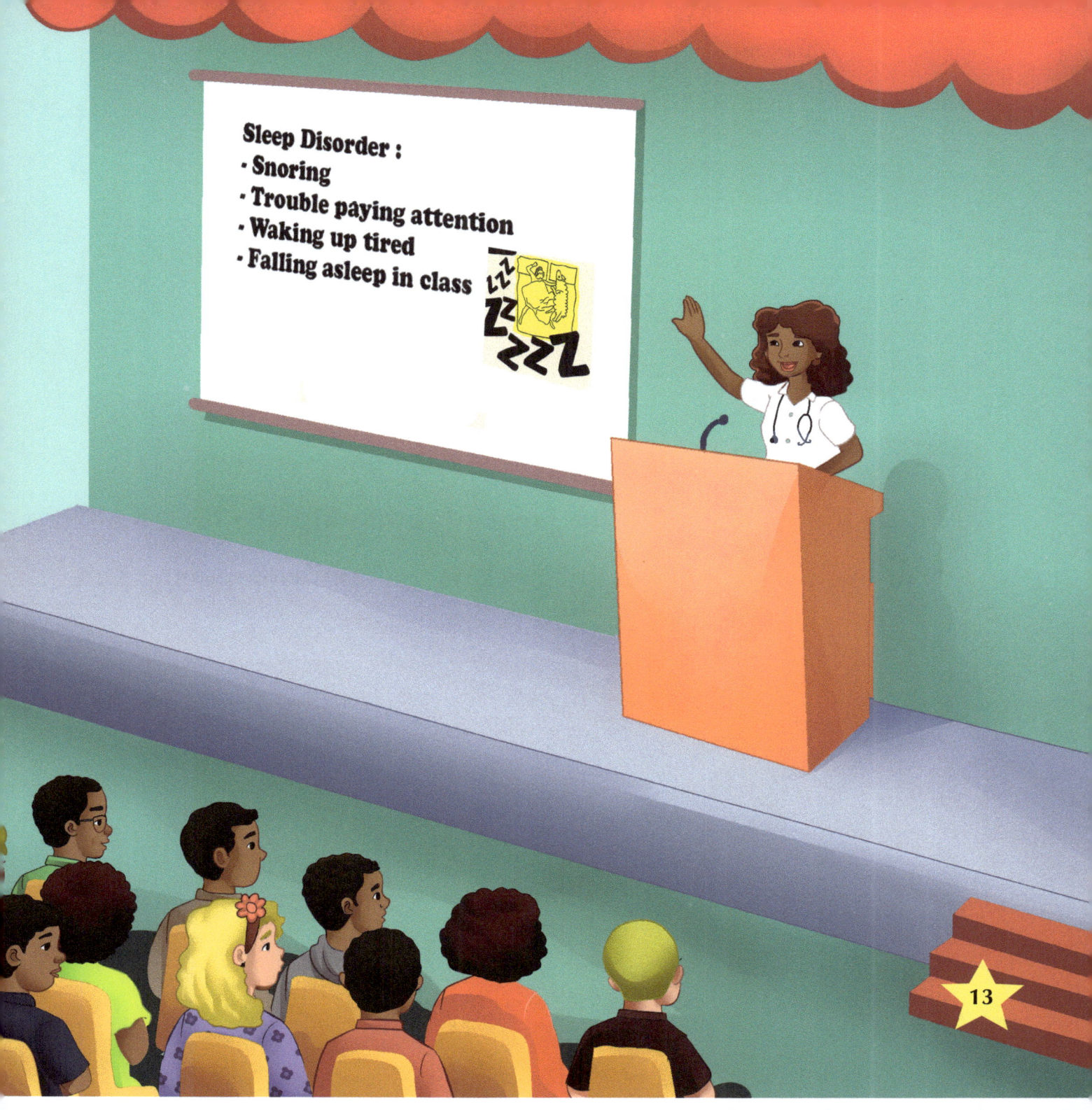

That night, Christopher told his mom everything.

About the doctor's talk. The poster. The snoring. The tired days.

"I'm really proud of you for speaking up," she said, pulling him into a hug.

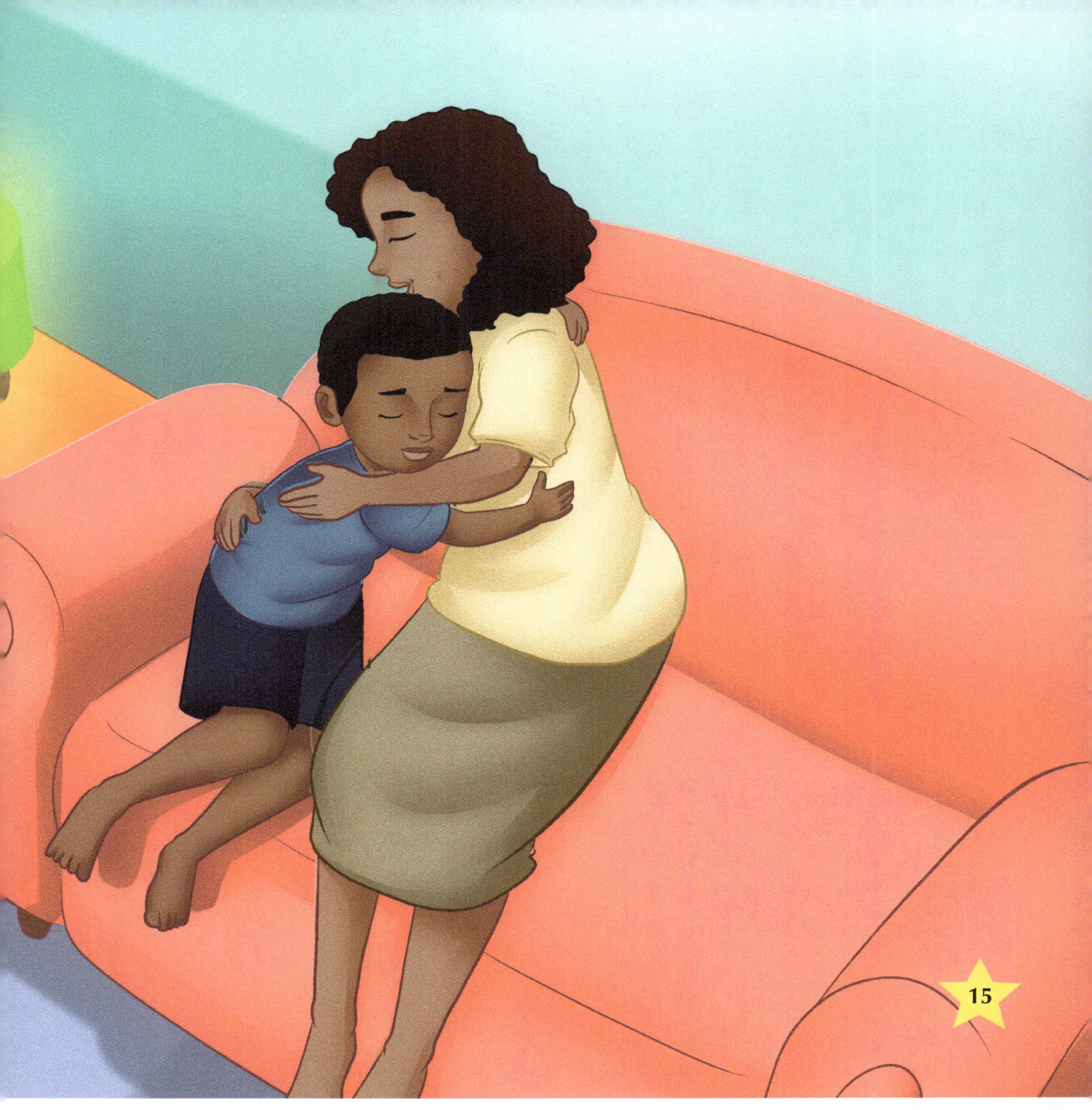

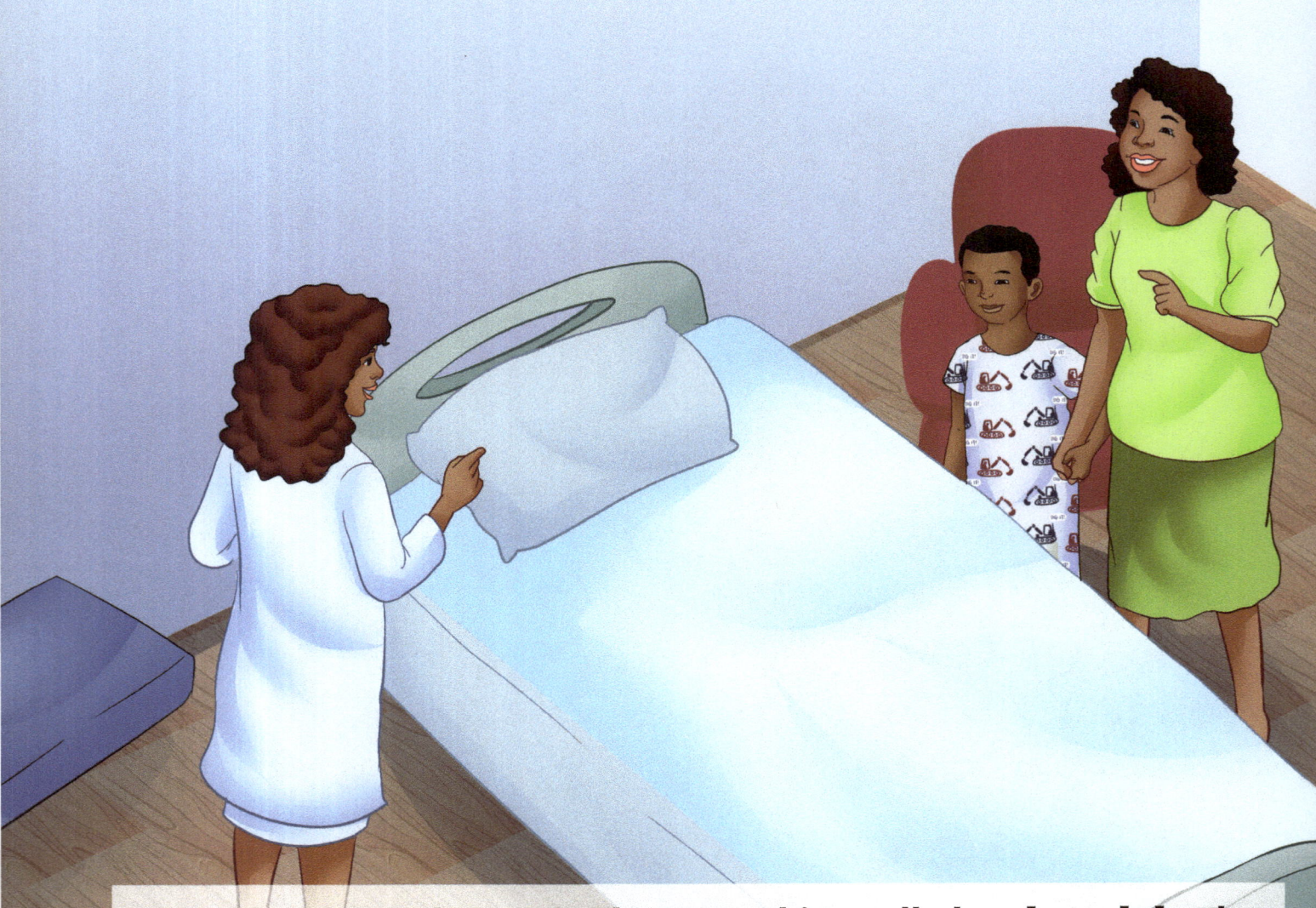

A few days later, they arrived to something called **a sleep lab**. The room looked like a cozy hotel with wood floors, a big soft bed, and even a little TV. There was a couch where his mom would sleep and a comfy chair in the corner.

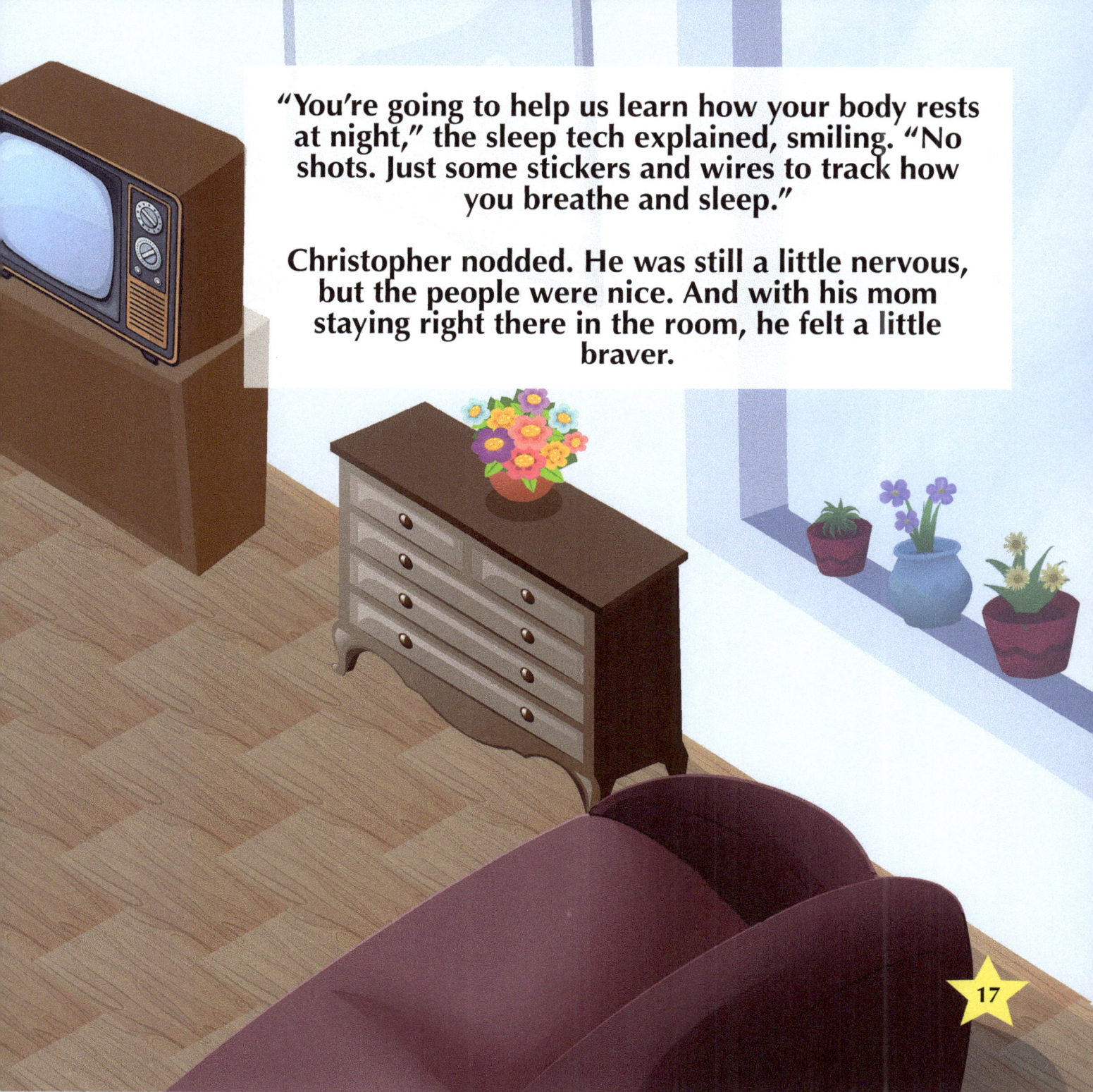

"You're going to help us learn how your body rests at night," the sleep tech explained, smiling. "No shots. Just some stickers and wires to track how you breathe and sleep."

Christopher nodded. He was still a little nervous, but the people were nice. And with his mom staying right there in the room, he felt a little braver.

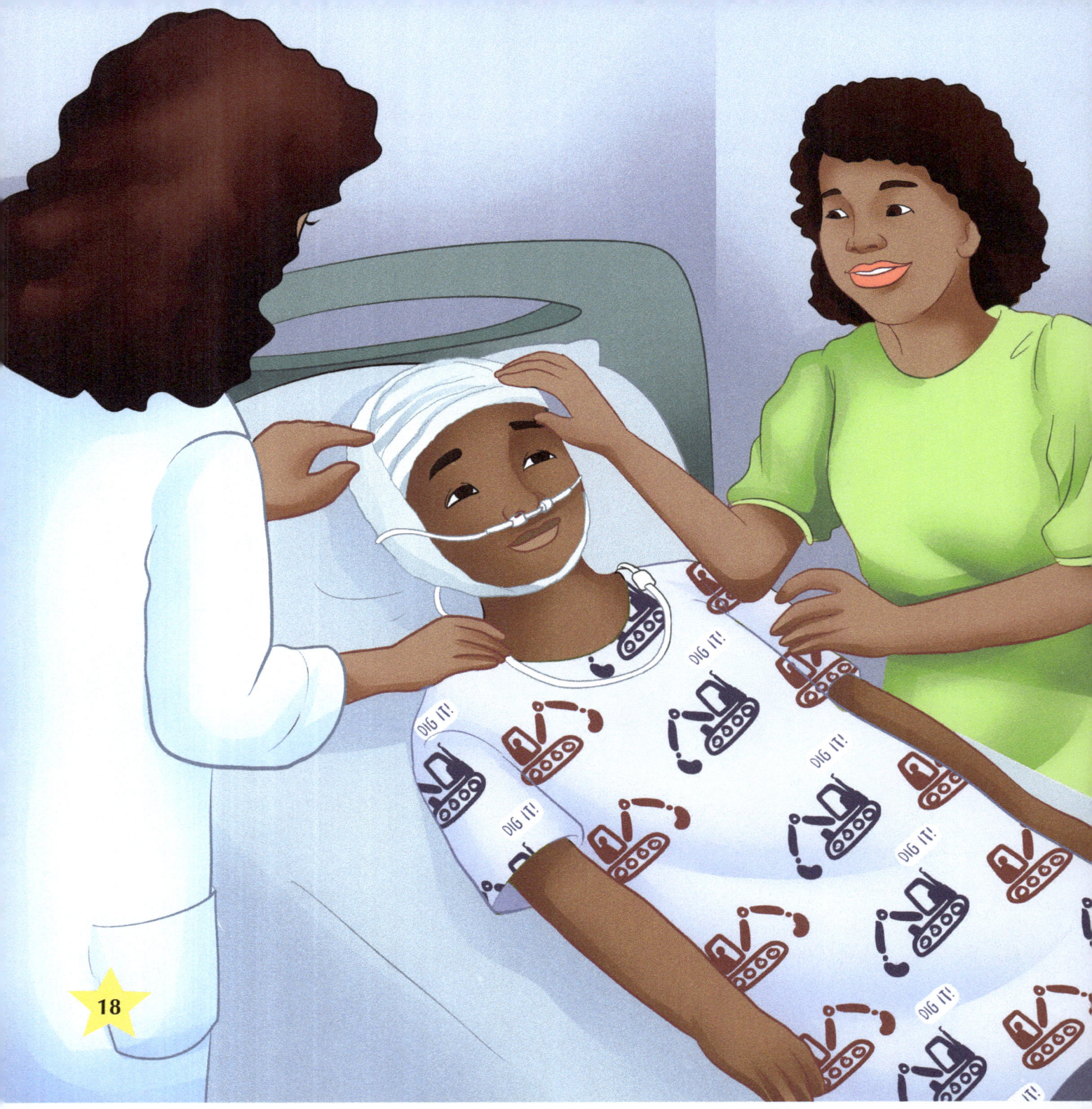

Getting ready for the study felt like an adventure. The technician gently placed soft stickers on Christopher's head, chest, and legs. They were connected to tiny wires that would watch how his body moved, breathed, and slept.
"You look like a robot," his mom teased, and they both laughed.

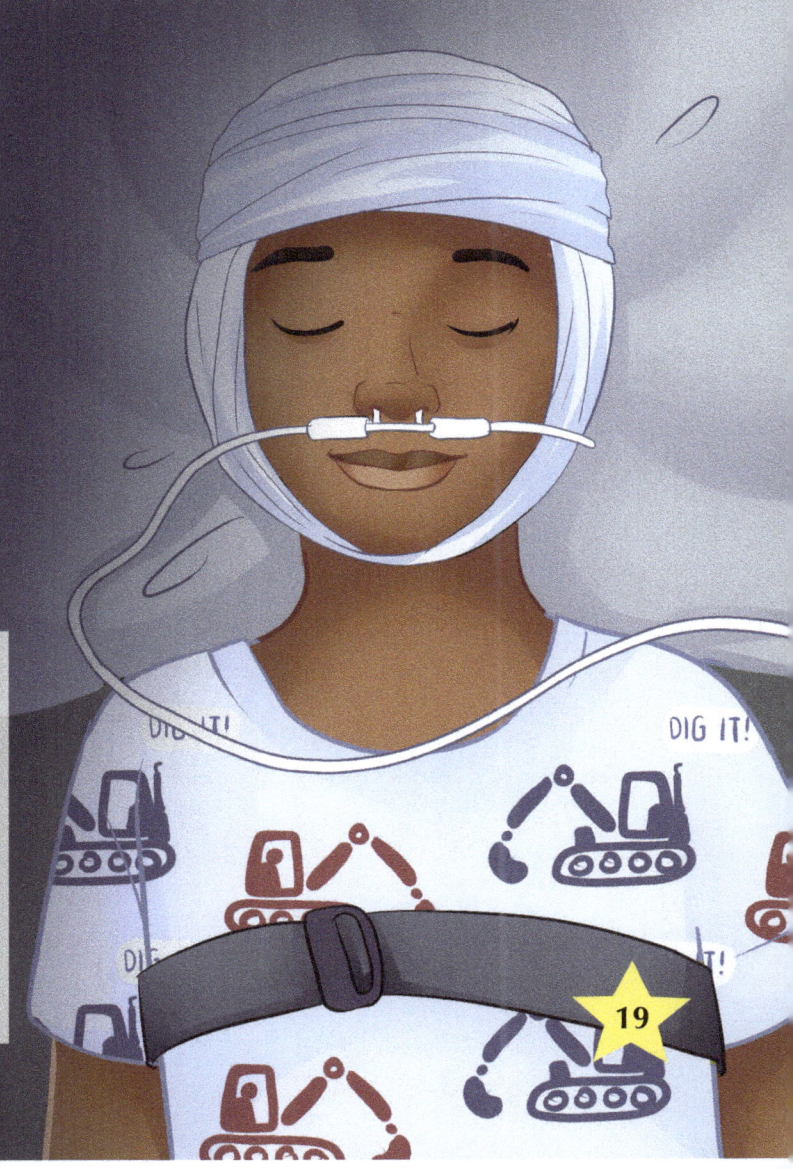

Once the lights were off, Christopher laid in bed, listening to the quiet hum of machines.

He wasn't sure if he'd fall asleep, but after a bedtime story and a goodnight hug from his mom, he drifted off.

A few days later, Christopher and his mom sat with the sleep doctor.

"You have something called **obstructive sleep apnea**," she explained kindly. "It means your breathing gets blocked sometimes when you sleep. That's why you snore and feel off during the day."

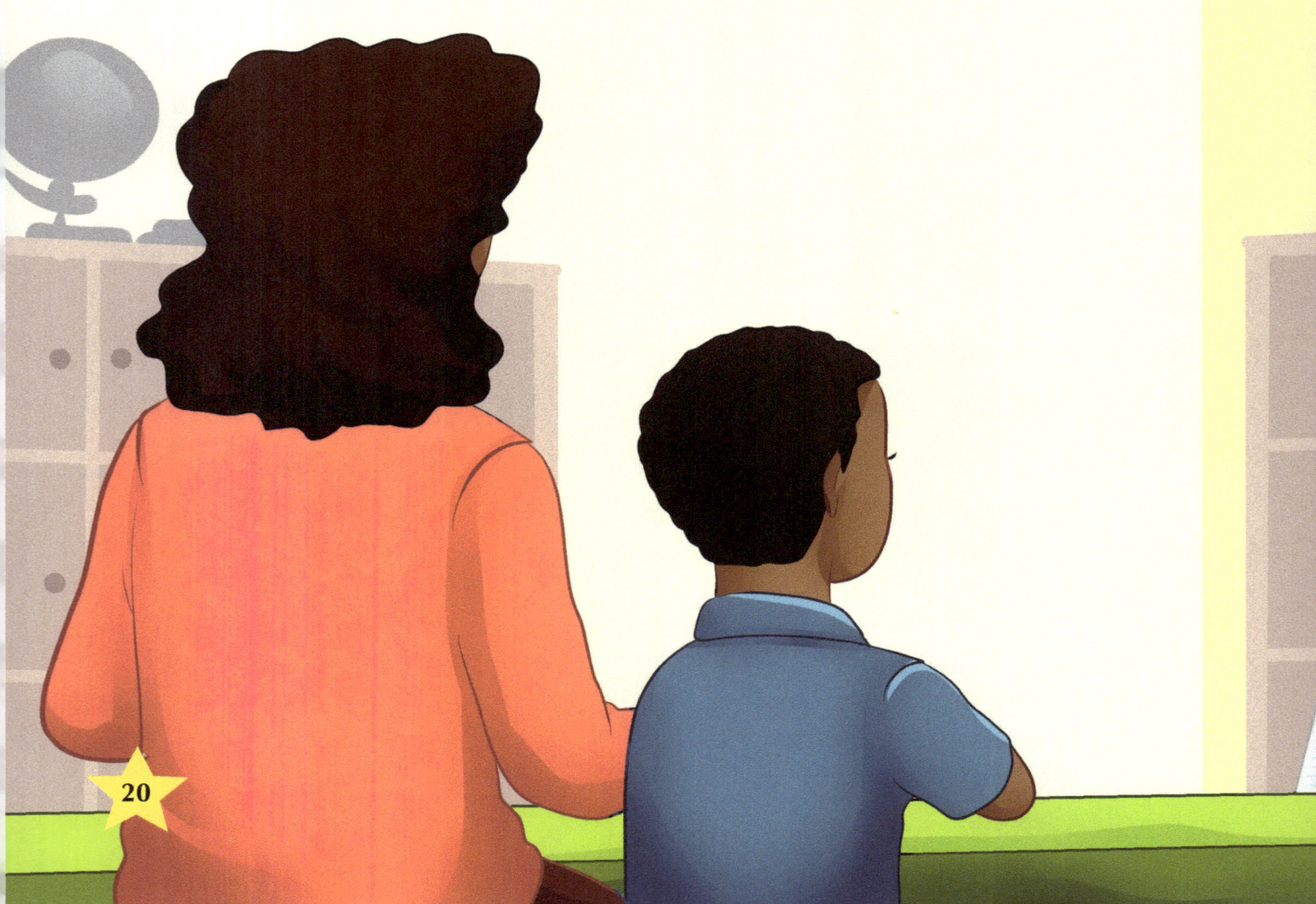

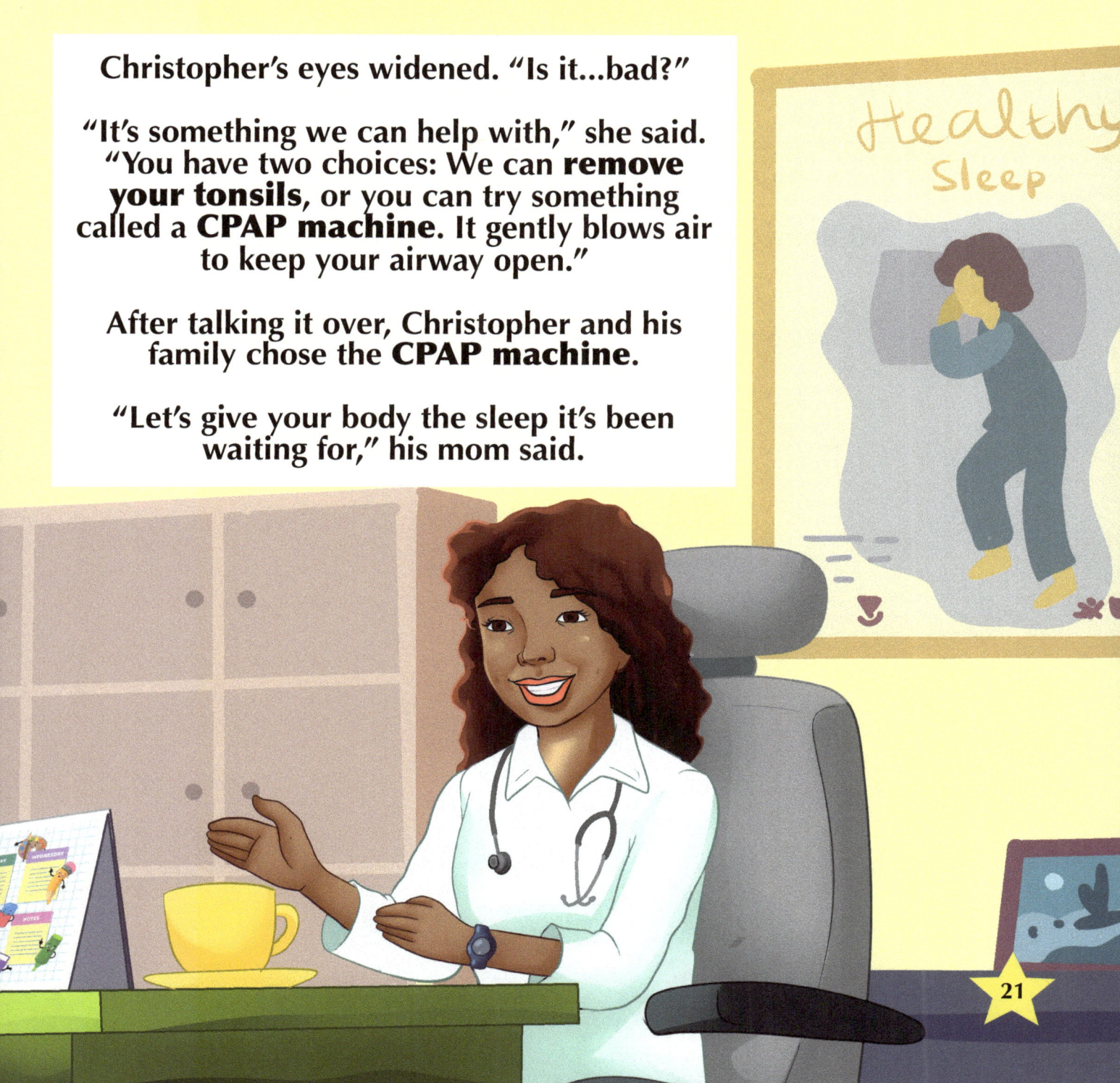

Christopher's eyes widened. "Is it...bad?"

"It's something we can help with," she said. "You have two choices: We can **remove your tonsils**, or you can try something called a **CPAP machine**. It gently blows air to keep your airway open."

After talking it over, Christopher and his family chose the **CPAP machine**.

"Let's give your body the sleep it's been waiting for," his mom said.

The first night with the **CPAP mask** felt...different.

The mask was soft and snug, with a small hose that gently puffed air into his nose while he slept.

At home, his family made a fun bedtime routine.

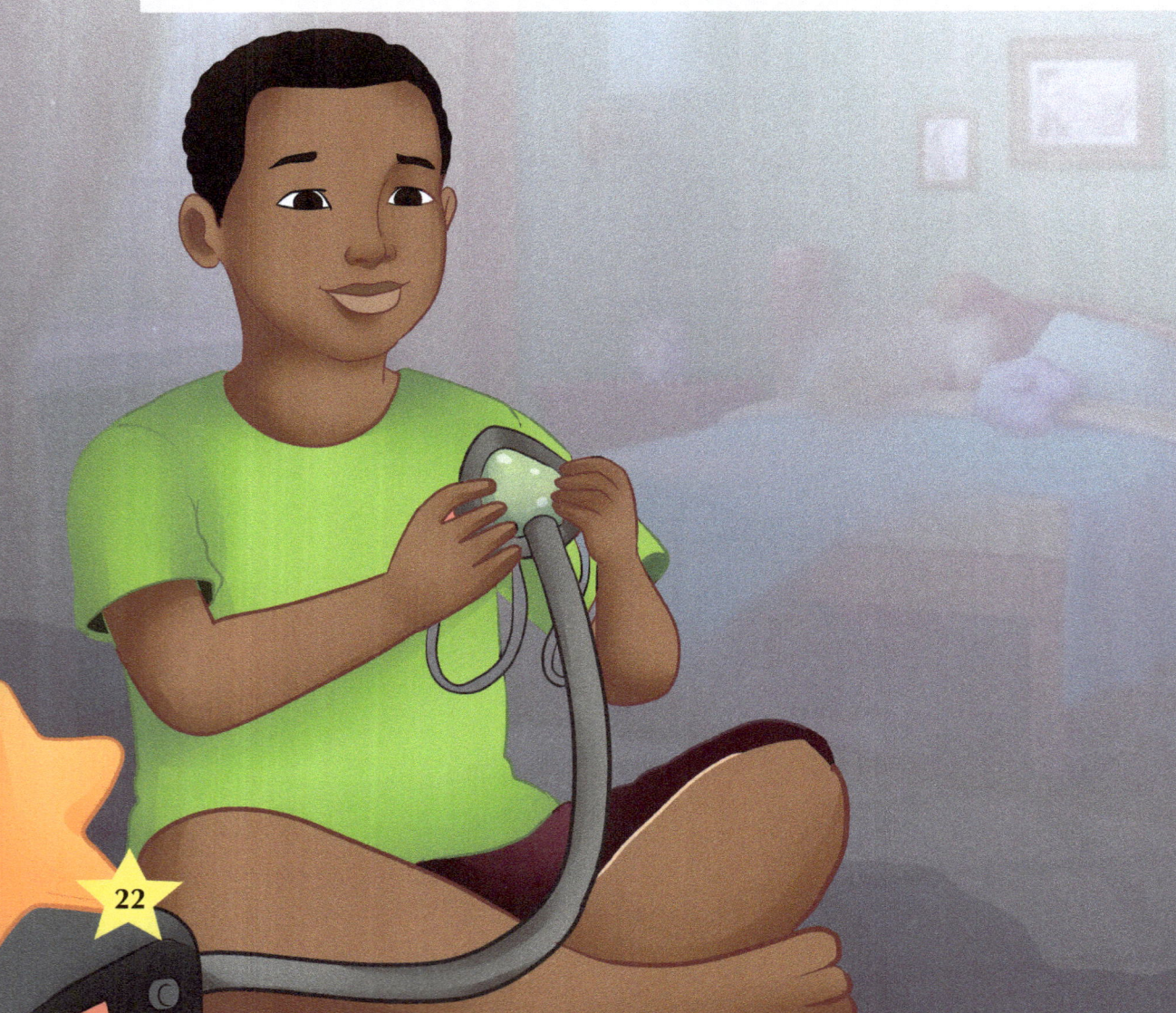

They named his machine **"Captain Puff."**

His sister decorated his mask with stickers.

Every night, his mom read him a story, tucked him in, and whispered, **"Sweet dreams."**

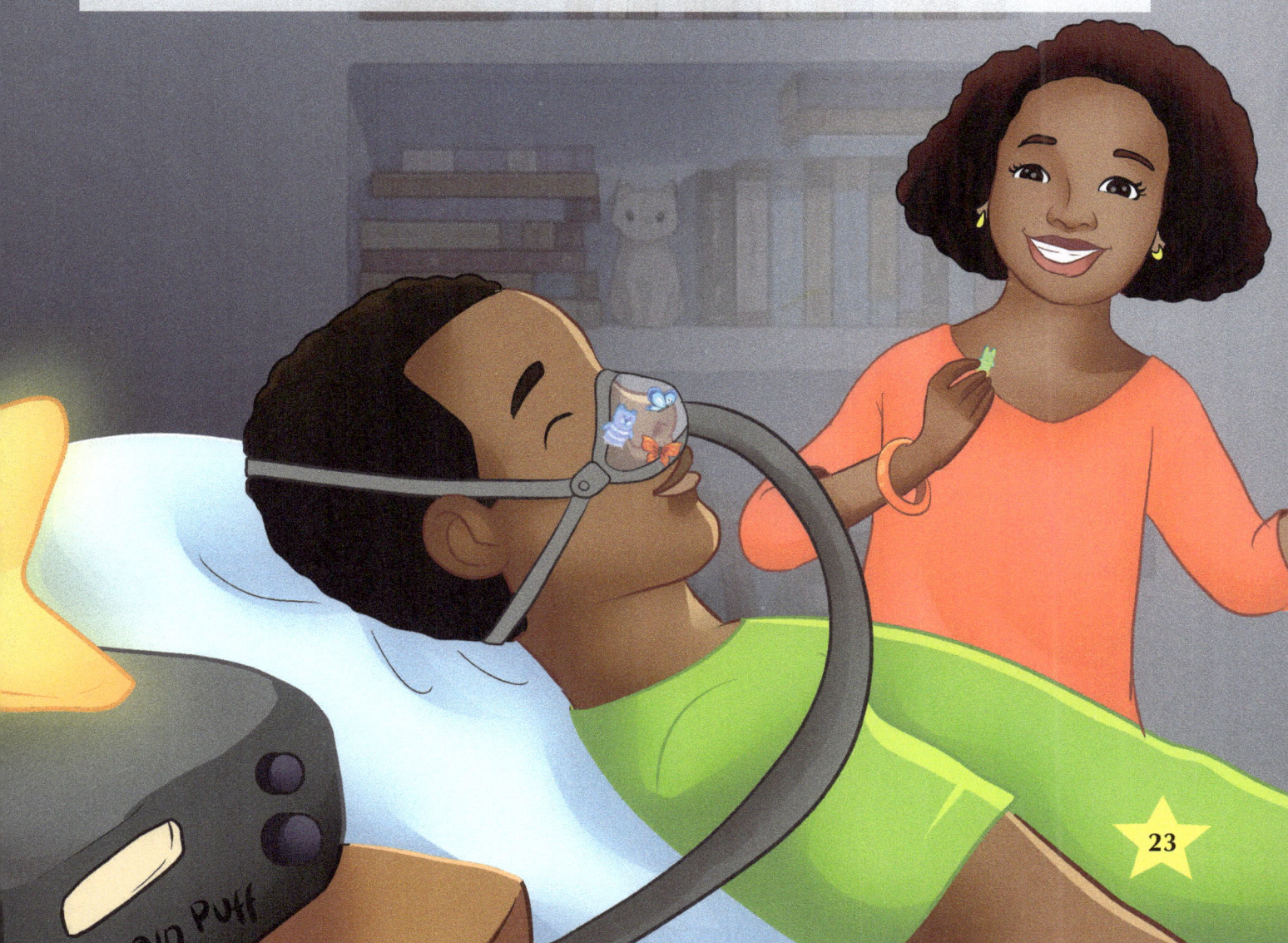

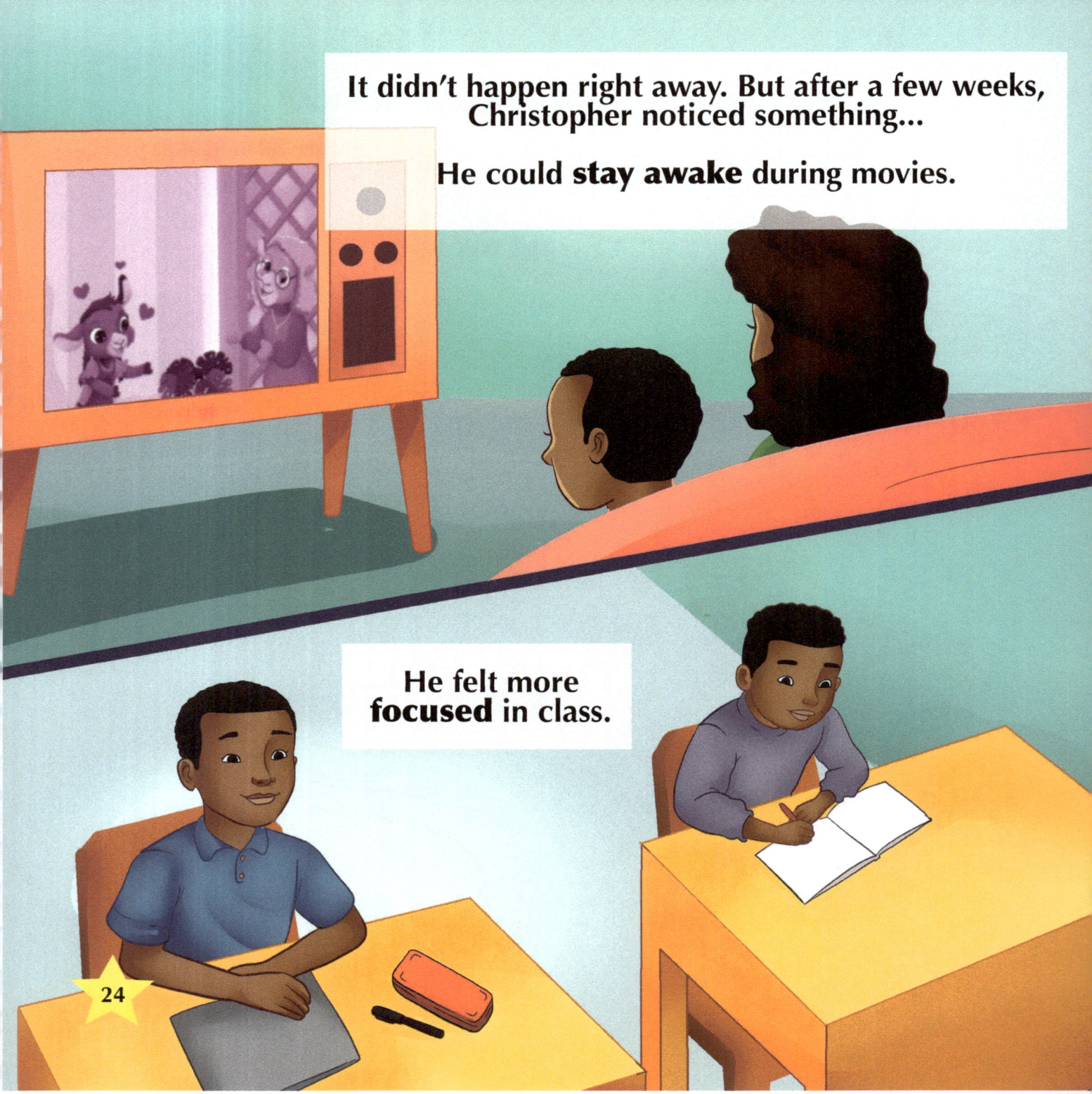

And on long road trips with his great-grandparents, he stayed awake the whole time.

"You're like a new person," his great-grandma smiled.

"There's my co-pilot," his great-grandfather said. "Couldn't have made it through Indiana without you."

Best of all?
No more teasing.
No more snoring.

Christopher grinned wide. **"I feel like me!"**

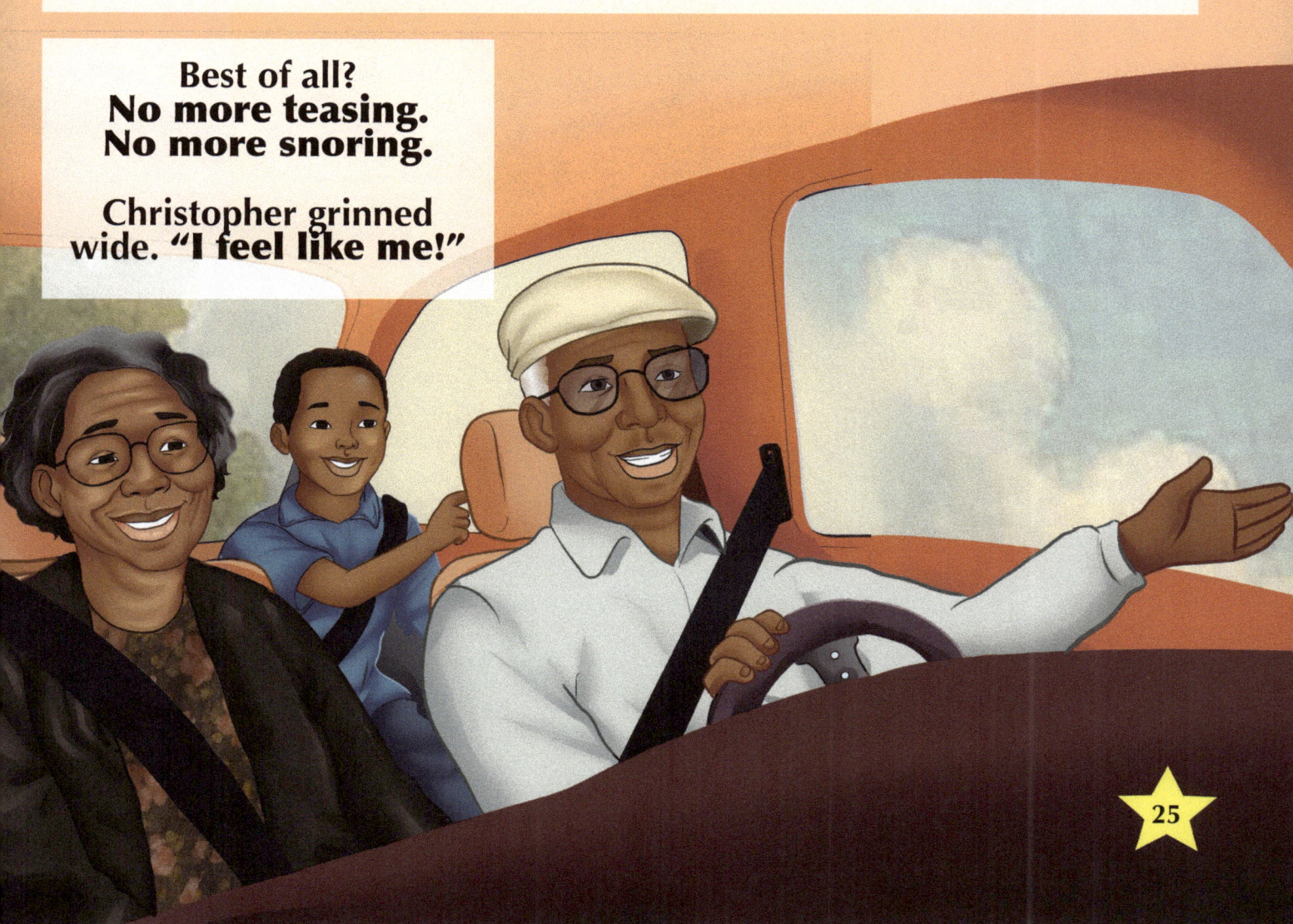

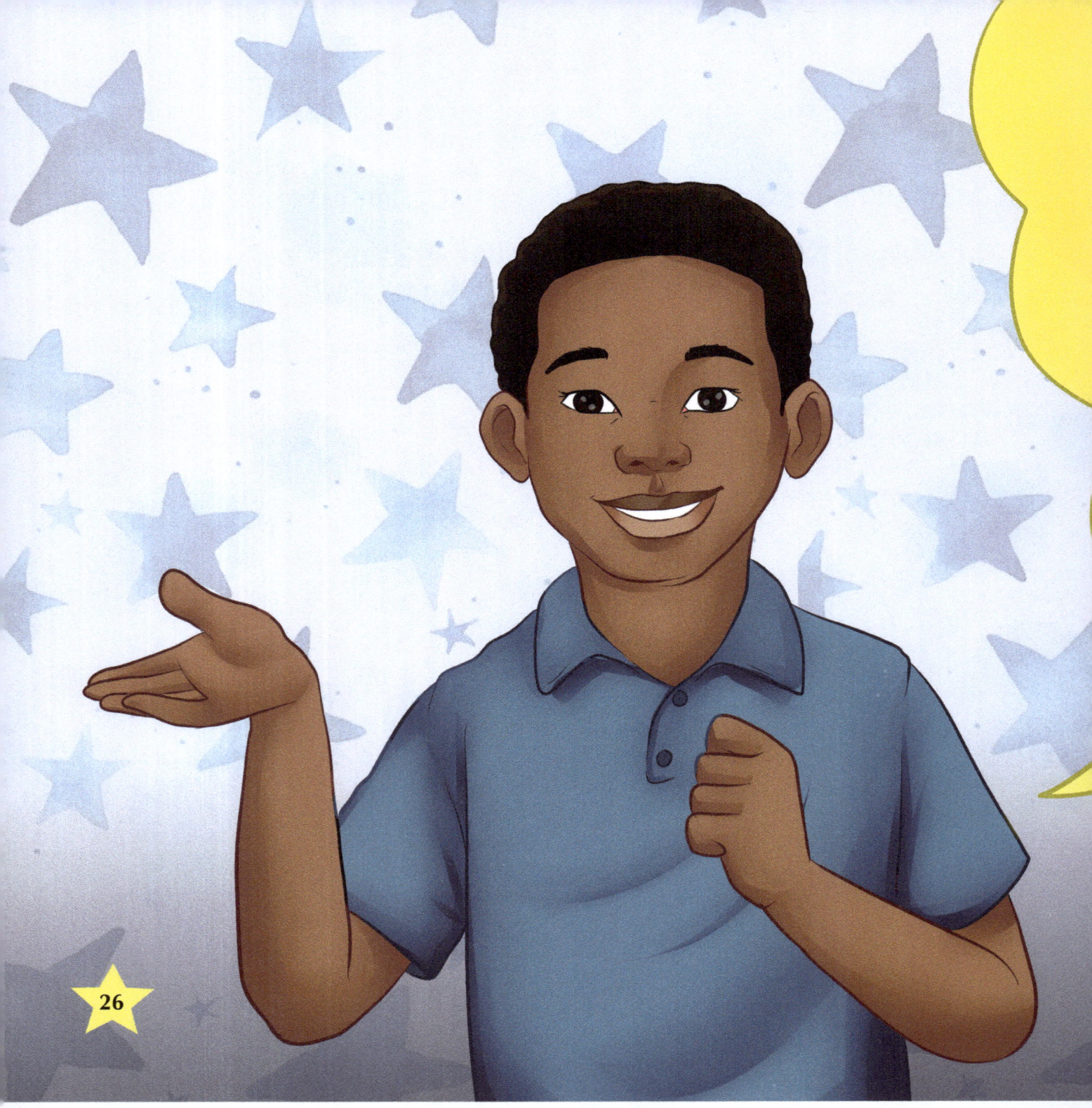

Christopher wants you to know something important:

"If you feel off, or people say you snore a lot, or you're always tired-even when you sleep - it's okay to talk about it. Tell a parent, a teacher, or a doctor. You might have a sleep disorder, just like I did. And if you do? You're not alone. There's help. There's hope. And there's rest waiting for you."

**Because sleep isn't just about bedtime.
Sleep helps you grow.
Sleep helps you focus.
Sleep helps you feel more like you.**

That night, after brushing his teeth and setting **"Captain Puff"** by his bed, Christopher looked out the window.

The stars were twinkling. His body felt calm. His mind felt clear.

He took one deep breath...
Then whispered into the night,
"Sweet dreams."

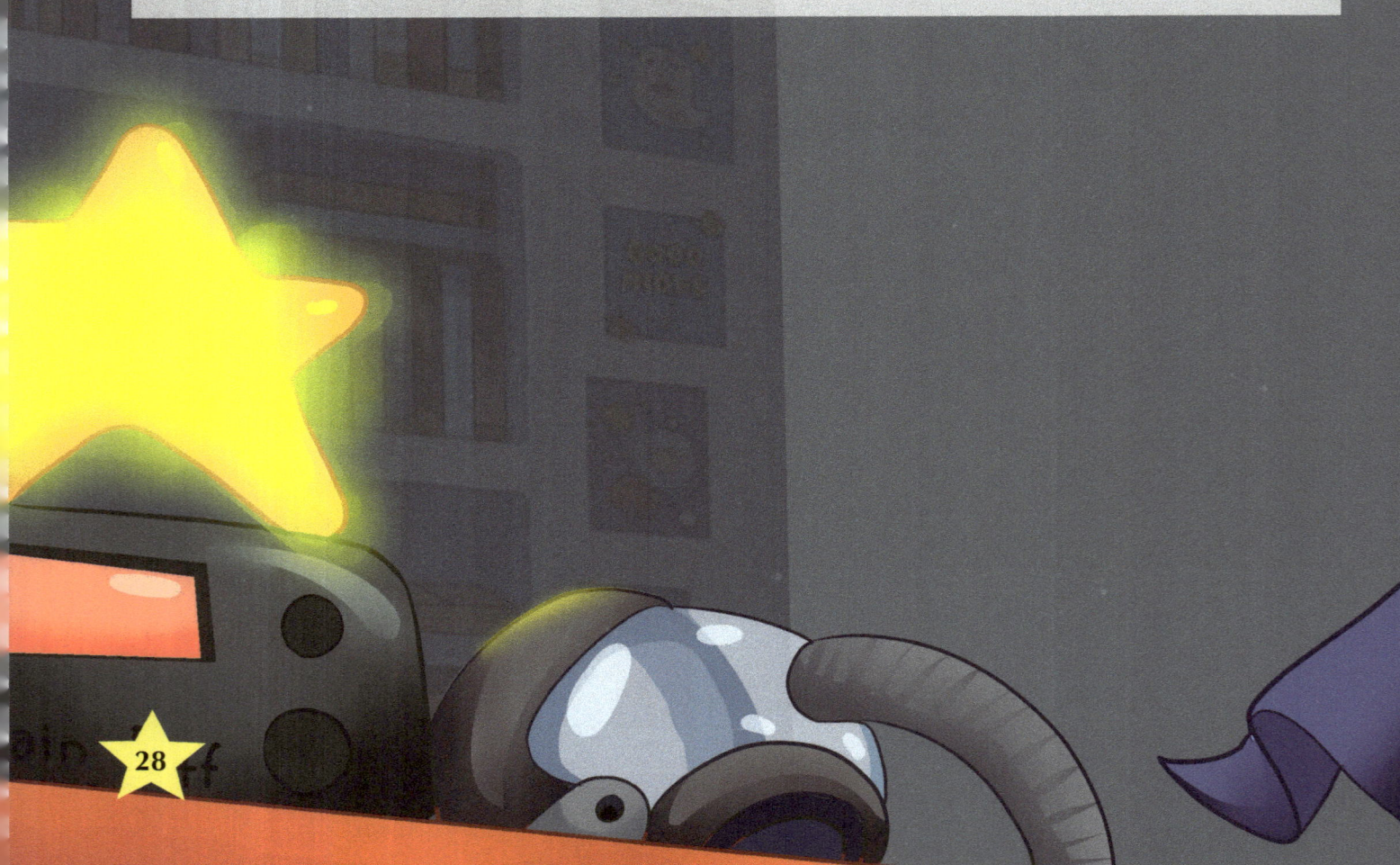

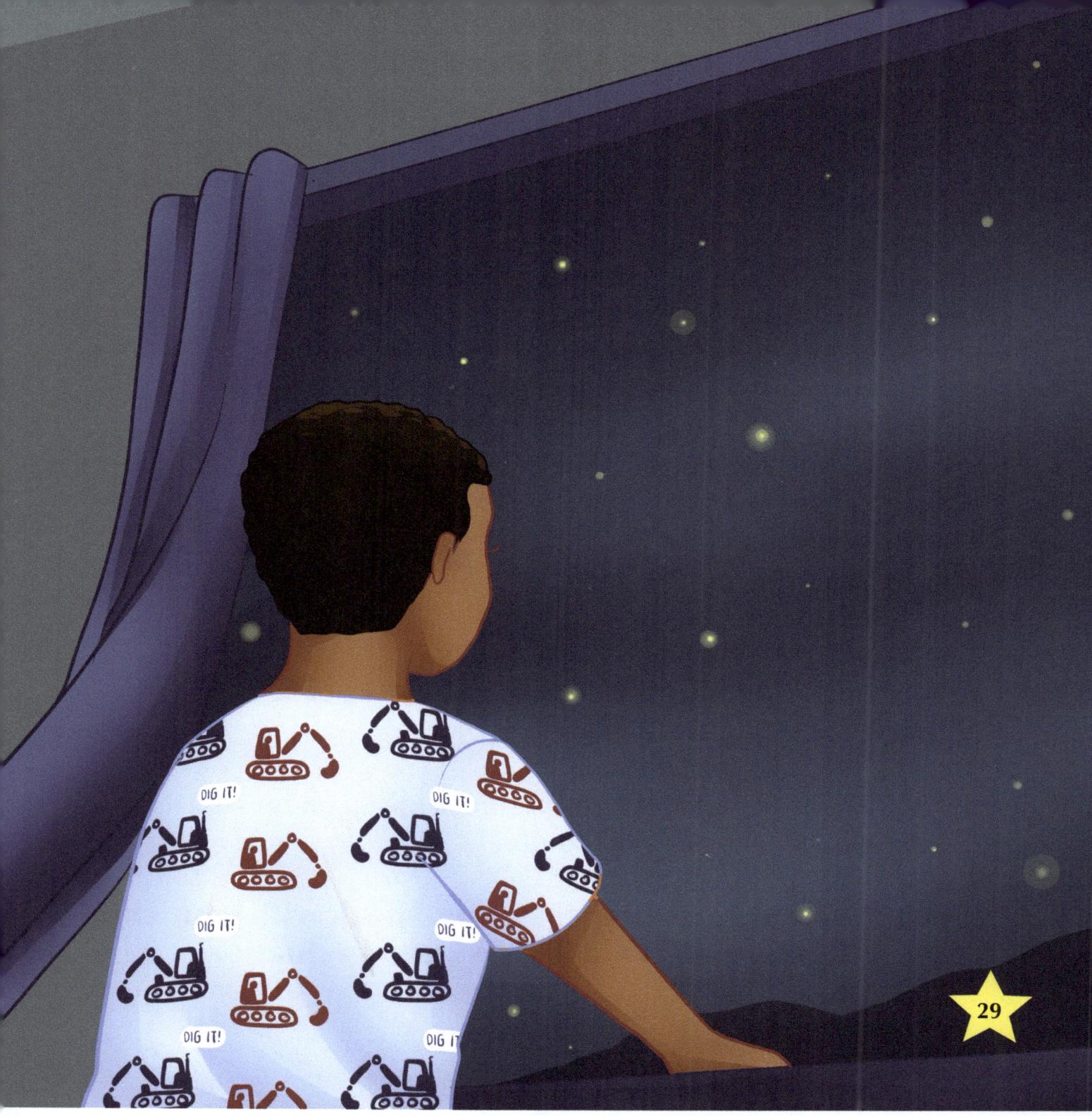

Parent & Caregiver Note:

Thank you for reading *Sweet Dreams* with your child.

Sleep is one of the most important-and most overlooked-parts of a child's health. Just like Christopher in this story, many children with sleep disorders go undiagnosed for years. But with early recognition and treatment, we can help them thrive.

Signs of Obstructive Sleep Apnea (OSA) in Children:

- Loud, frequent snoring
- Mouth breathing during sleep
- Pauses in breathing or gasping sounds
- Restless sleep or frequent awakenings
- Bedwetting (especially if it returns after being dry)
- Daytime sleepiness or fatigue
- Trouble focusing in school
- Moodiness or hyperactivity (sometimes mistaken for ADHD)
- Morning headaches or dry mouth

If you notice several of these signs, speak with your child's doctor about a possible sleep evaluation.

Recommended Sleep Duration by Age:

- 3-5 years: 10-13 hours (including naps)
- 6-12 years: 9-12 hours
- 13-18 years: 8-10 hours

Every child deserves restful sleep-and a bright, energized day ahead.

For more support, visit **www.SleepDrChris.com** and **www.qualitysleepandneurology.com** or follow **@SleepDrChris** for more tips on healthy sleep.

32

Acknowledgements

To my family, my patients, and every parent who stays up late making sure their children get the rest they need. This book is for you.

And to the children who see themselves in Christopher: your story matters, and your dreams are worth protecting.

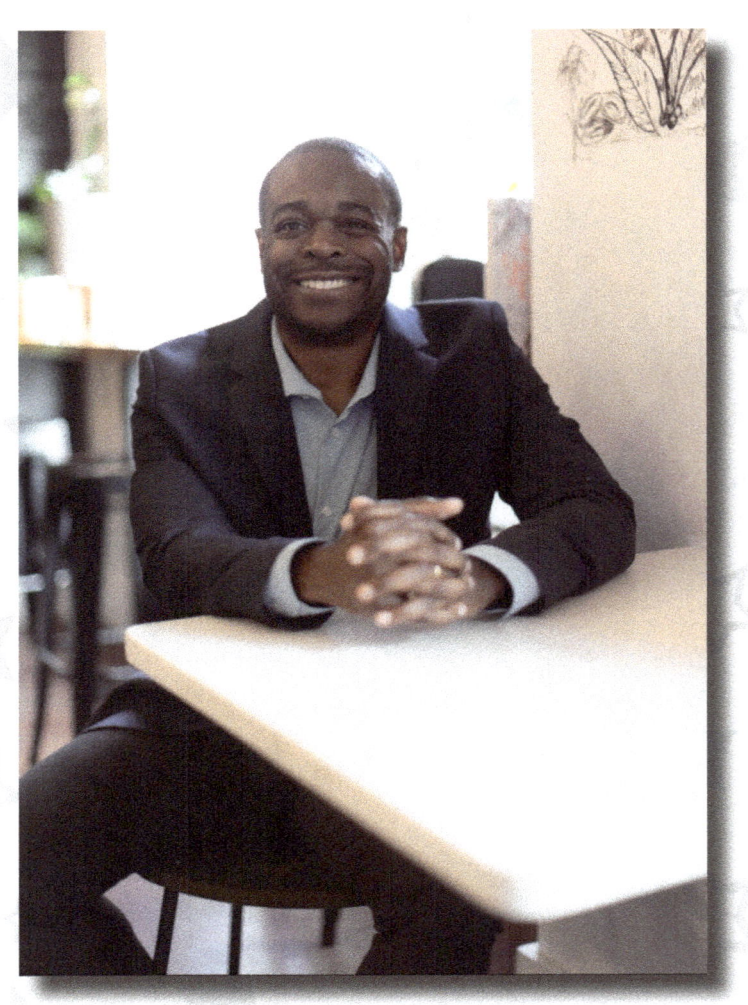

Dr. Christopher J. Allen is a board-certified pediatric neurologist and sleep medicine doctor, and the founder of Quality Sleep and Neurology PC.

He was inspired to write *Sweet Dreams* by his own experience with obstructive sleep apnea and the life-changing difference treatment made for him.

Today, Dr. Allen helps children and families understand that sleep is not just rest — it's healing. Through his practice, speaking engagements, and online platform **@SleepDrChris**, he continues to educate and empower others to make sleep a priority.

When he's not caring for patients or creating content, Dr. Allen enjoys traveling with his family and making memories with his wife and two children.

105 Publishing LLC
www.105publishing.com
Austin, TX

www.ingramcontent.com/pod-product-compliance
Lightning Source LLC
Chambersburg PA
CBHW040001040426
42337CB00032B/5180